Table for Two
Dining with Dementia

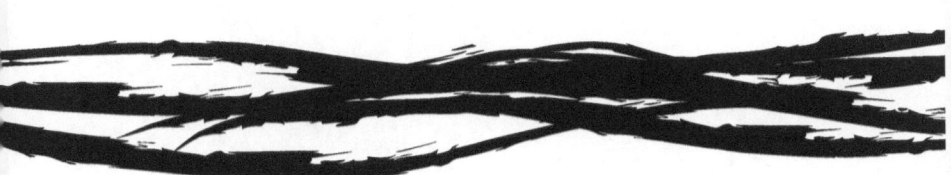

Kimberlee Alsup

*A caregiver's guide
to making mealtime great*

ISBN: 1-4392-1841-2
ISBN-13: 9781439218419

Visit www.booksurge.com to order additional copies.

For questions about information in this book, contact the author at
delectables4u@hotmail.com

TABLE OF CONTENTS

INTRODUCTION

Life today is a very fast paced phenomenon. We hustle and hurry to complete this and that. We try to keep up with our to-do lists in ways that we are convinced makes us whole and complete. But for a person with memory impairment, there is an eroding and subtle influence affecting the ability to control things in life. Those tasks at hand can seem overwhelming. The list may be made yet the ability to carry it out has evaporated. For you, the caregiver, the list grows, and for the memory impaired, the list is now the enemy. It is with this very compassion for the environment we call life that surrounds the memory impaired and their caregiver that this book is written.

Not many folks truly understand what it takes to care for a person with dementia until they are smack in the middle of the situation, with little preparation, some with no experience at all, and the daunting task of making sense of the world for this individual who is grasping at threads of recall, trying to process everyday events with all the energy they can muster. So as time marches forward in this role, the care given to the afflicted person can range from low-key housekeeping and meal preparation, to full-fledged figuring everything out for two, all day long.

As demanding and tall as this order may be, the object of this book is to lighten the load for the caregiver of a memory impaired person, especially where food is concerned. We have many classes and books on how to bath, dress, medicate, treat wounds, and nurse. Not yet have I come across a real hands-on manual for how to address the largest and most important part of every human's world – the food we eat, and what it means to us.

As you peruse Table for Two, do so with the understanding that the caregiver is the person who needs the most support when it comes to food. This is the reason for the book. Preserving our past, through food, by making every meal matter, is the heart and soul of this edition.

While reading this book, you may realize that you would like to take many of the questions and apply them to your life, and creating your own food story. For it is by learning the puzzles of the memory impaired that we find their joy and create a newfound world for them, by reclaiming their rich past and celebrating their precious lives.

Bringing together the insights of years of hands-on experience as a cook, a supporter to caregivers, a problem-greeter and a trouble-shooter, the intent here is to recollect for you, the caregiver, the precious time and energy that escapes you on a daily basis. This book is meant to give you the answers you may be looking for in helping the memory impaired person to get the most out of their meal experience, while giving you the breathing room that you need. Caregiving is not for sissies- so buckle up and get ready for a ride on the dementia dining express!

CHAPTER 1

REASONS WE EAT:
THE CONNECTIONS ARE UNIQUE

As we journey together though this discussion about food and dementia care, it is so important to convey that each caregiver has a very unique set of circumstances, along with a very unique individual that they have the responsibility of caring for. This book by no means claims or supposes to answer every question and concern that might arise. Rather, this book intends to provide a basis for establishing a personal dining 'care plan,' if you will. Within the basic parameters you will learn, there is the hope that your creative talents and insights will blend with the thoughts and stories here to accomplish a new and successful style of care.

For the purposes of this book, the terms that are used have been applied somewhat interchangeably, namely that a person with memory impairment will parallel to the description of a person with dementia. Since the term 'dementia' is thought of as a broad umbrella for any set of symptoms that present as cognitive decline (or memory impairment), the terms are used to describe the same individual.

The memory decline diagnosis, whether specified as Alzheimer's Disease, vascular dementia, frontal temporal dementia, Lewy-Body dementia, or a host of other dementias, will inevitably become a progressive condition. To help with easing the decline of the dementia, the aspect of nutrition, through proper meal preparation and a host of other elements you will discover, becomes paramount to achieving a higher quality of life. From eating properly to stave off illness, to keeping the brain functioning as well as possible, the more awareness we have on how food intake affects our bodies and general health, the better.

In an attempt to help make the caregiving day go smoother, there are countless activities, tasks and simple measures that, when applied, can ease the load of the day. Once a strategy has been formed to meet meals with open hearts and minds, we can creatively involve the memory impaired person in ways that are rewarding and meaningful for all concerned. Our task then becomes finding the right strategy for our situation.

In my 12 years of experience with persons of all stages and levels of dementia, I have had the very personal honor of working with those who come from all walks of life, from many different cultures and backgrounds, and with a generation that existed many years before I was born. The pleasure and enrichment I have received from these individuals, their families and friends, has been inconceivable. This most rewarding pleasure, of assisting in and contributing to improve the quality of life for all, be it for a short while or for many years during the disease process, has led me to the pinnacle of sharing these experiences in my hope to bless others.

A personal gift in this work for me has been the numerous nuggets of wisdom that have been imparted to me through those I have worked with. The amazing element of memory I have witnessed is the ability a person with dementia has to recall, ever so vividly, events, stories, experiences, tastes and flavors of the distant past. Sitting with someone who can reminisce so clearly about their 11th birthday party – who was present, what happened, what kind of cake they had, and the gifts that came that day – never ceases to amaze me. To learn so much by conversation such as this is like a precious gift that will be stored forever in my heart.

For you and your memory impaired person, I wish the great gift of sharing time, experiences and wisdom together. For it is through these experiences, that we all learn to connect at a deeper level than ever imagined. For you I wish this gift of love.

While creating a dining care plan can be a gratifying exercise, the work is never completely finished with a memory impaired person. Due to the ever-changing abilities, ranging from mental to physical to emotional to psychological, our mission is to try to keep the constant of food and its pleasures ever in front of the curve. When this occurs, the person has a much better opportunity to live a life with pleasure and delight.

To begin to understand the person with dementia, as it relates to food, we must reflect upon our own set of values that are formed. Beginning at a very young age, we want nourishment, which then equates to pleasure, and then the motives can run in 264 directions – sometimes many directions all at once. By the time we've reached adulthood, our tastes have developed for certain foods, we have routines we covet, and we 'dine' in many different styles. The food and mealtime values you form may differ completely from those food values that I form.

The reasons we eat are as varied and layered and unique as every individual that walks this earth. Every person alive has their own set of very intimate food preferences, connections, memories, habits, and traditions. We all relate to food in a very personal way. It is a wonder that we actually sit down and enjoy the same meal together, once we realize the makeup we each bring to the table.

We know that there are common threads within people that help us to come to recognize patterns, Our customs, culture and generational values bring many aspects of our lifestyle together. We can see the results of this very clearly. However, there is a basic blend of attributes to our food value systems that can be identified as the social, emotional and physical. These three areas of value-building create in each of us a personal perspective toward our most basic need.

SOCIAL DINING

Since the beginning of time, we eat gather and gain sustenance together. We hunt, cultivate, fish, harvest, cook, and sup together. We gain nourishment in what we call community. The coming together and breaking of bread as a group.

This classic model is seen in the large Italian families. You must eat together, all 15 of you at once. The meal is not the meal without Uncle Louie and Aunt Reggie from next door there. And where is second cousin Anthony? (...He must be coming, so we shall wait...)

Another aspect of social dining is that of the retired couple who has taken every meal together for 49 years. They would not think of sitting down to a meal alone. It just can't happen.

Also, we come together at family celebrations, to cheer on the birthday boy, or to toast the anniversary of Tom and Jane. These times make food more meaningful and make for lifelong memories.

When we think of special occasions, food becomes the centerpiece, and the momentum builds until the carving tools come out and the turkey is sliced. We pass bowls and gravy boats as a celebration of unity over a day of remembrance. We toast to the good times, cheer the newlyweds, and give thanks for our many blessings. These are all rich memories that are stored deep within the soul.

Dining out for some people has been a big part of their lives. Restaurant after restaurant, some have had the luxury of being waited on for more meals than not. For some, the experience of meeting new people at restaurants, or attending dinner parties and upscale affairs has been their way of connecting, with food as the secondary reason for gathering.

EMOTIONAL EATING

Food can create intimate connections in our being, the way nothing else can. We learn as infants to connect emotionally, and we react when we don't get what we want, when we want it. As we age, our comfort level with food grows to a more prominent level than ever before in our lives. We cling to food memories that beckon back to days gone by. Our mind takes us back to vanilla ice cream served over grandma's homemade apple pie, just out of the oven. Before we know it, we are tasting that pie, needing that pie, and needing grandma, too.

Many people have such strong emotional ties to food, that food becomes their comfort all through their lives, especially during ANY emotional occasion! Feeling bored, let's eat...feeling happy, let's eat...feeling sad or stressed,... let's definitely eat!

As we go through life, we have bonded to certain foods that hold an emotional connection, deeper than the food itself. Remember your favorite dish that mom always made for you on your birthday? Yes, I bet you do. And you would enjoy having it just about anytime, right?

For many people, food becomes their best friend. It will always satisfy, ease pain, support, make you smile and feel loved. No wonder we are impulsive eaters, we want to feel good - always!

PHYSICAL NEEDS

This might seem like the most obvious reason we eat. But for a person with dementia, this becomes the area of *least* concern. When time relationships become distorted, so does the body clock. Your memory impaired person may already be experiencing the effects of an unwound body clock: restless and sleepless nights, mixing up day with night, sleeping during the day, and other signs.

We get our energy, vitality, nutrition, hydration and replenish our bodies through food. How can we live without if? We can't.

Because food provides the mainstay of our existence, we have to have it. We especially depend on the calories we receive for our energy supply and our well being. Did you know that a person that has a low carbohydrate level could become increasingly confused? Carbohydrates are the main food source the brain uses to function. Without adequate carbs, our heads are foggy and faint. Our thinking patterns are less clear and we may experience lapses in recall. These are all important signals to remember when giving care to a person with dementia.

As you may now see, we each have built a very complex story of why we eat, when we eat, how we eat, what we eat, and who eats with us. How can we make sense of the values that are built inside the person with memory impairment? We know that there are reasons tucked inside each person, whether they can articulate them or not. It might not even be an option to ask, but someone, somewhere in their past, can lend insights into the values you hope to learn.

By now you might be asking yourself why we are discussing psychological concepts surrounding food values. What about the help that you need to make mealtime successful?

Follow me, if you will, and we will embark on a food journey that just may answer this question, and may offer you a game plan to get started.

CHAPTER 2

THE ROLE PLAY OF FOOD

Now that we have seen how food connections are so very special for every person, we have a new sense of how important it is to make sure we are taking these personal values into account. Often, a caregiver may not know about the food connections someone has, nor is the memory impaired person able to express their values. This is when we rely on family members, friends and neighbors – those close to the person – to help us uncover these connections.

When you enlist the help of others that know your person, especially long-time friends and older family members (siblings are a great help), the information you can glean is priceless. To learn about this person's past, in a food-sense, can open so many doorways, and provide a plentiful supply of kitchen 'tools' to use, for countless days to come. Besides the opportunity to provide enrichment and reconnection to the past, we are tapping into emotional memories that help the mind to reminisce. This is helpful, healthy, and very beneficial to the person with dementia.

So now it is time to do our detective work. Below are some questions you may find helpful to ask people who are close to the person with memory impairment. If the person you are trying to learn more about is able, ask the questions directly. It will be an honor and a compliment to them.

Does John come from a large family? A small family?

How many children does he have? Are there grandchildren, and if so, how many?

How has John celebrated holidays in the past? Which ones were his favorites?

What are some of John's favorite foods? Ask for past favorites and present favorites.

Does John sleep in or get up early?

What has John's life routine been like?

Is John a coffee shop kind of guy?

What does John traditionally like for break-fast?

What has been his favorite meal of the day?

What is his favorite beverage to drink?

Does John have any food allergies?

Does he prefer certain kinds of foods?

All these questions, and more like them that you may think up, are valuable in establishing a food story for the person you are caring for. I would encourage you to ask as many people close to John as possible - they can all lead you with different pieces of information that could make your food experiences with John much more enjoyable!

When we learn the patterns of a person with dementia, mealtime can clearly become a difference between night and day. Let me tell you a story:

Rose was a woman who was an early riser all her life. She was a farmer's wife, and her husband Don was up at 4:00 AM to start his day. Don would nudge her as he rolled out of bed, and then he proceeded to get dressed. Rose would wake a little slower, roll out of bed by 5:00 and prepare breakfast for Don as he was out in the barn, gearing up for his day of work. Rose would have his breakfast on the table by 5:30, they would eat, and start the day. Rose would then sit down with the radio on and do the dishes, humming along with the tune she was listening to. After that, Rose would take her bath and see after the household chores. Once Rose had started the laundry, swept the kitchen, watered the garden and fed the dogs, she would begin to prepare the large meal of the day, which in the Midwest, was at noontime, and was called **dinner.** This meal gave the men on the farm, husband and hired hands, the chance to fill their bellies and continue about their hard working day.

After the men returned to the field, Rose would clean up the kitchen and sit down to do either darning, mending, sewing, letter writing, or the like. The next activity was **suppertime,** which was much lighter than dinner and usually was served about 5:00 PM. consisting of a reheat from dinner with bread or crackers, fruit, and maybe pudding for dessert. Once the supper meal was over, the kitchen was cleaned again and the day was 'set to rest'. Reading or porch-sitting was the activity in order. Rose was then back in bed by 8:00 PM where she would rest and look to begin again the next day. This was the order of Rose's married life. Her routine was pretty much the same for the 42 years she was farming with Don.

FAST FORWARD TO PRESENT TIME:

Rose is now 82 years old and has been diagnosed with moderate level dementia. Rose needs someone to help her with her life tasks, from bathing to dressing to meal preparation. Rose mostly sits now, looking out the window as if she is waiting for something or someone. She is patient and calm most of the time, except for mid-morning and mid-afternoon. At these times she appears restless, will pace the house and fidget, sometimes getting into drawers, picking things up and looking confused. Rose has little speech activity, but will accept direction and can express herself when she wants to. Most of the time when meals are served, Rose comes to the table and stares blankly at the food as though she doesn't recognize it. She sometimes just watches while others eat. Sometimes she gets up, walks to the kitchen sink, and just stares out the window.

Why do I tell you this story? We find many clues in it that are very important to making Rose happy in her sunset years of life. As Rose's caregiver, there are many things that can be done to assist Rose in having a meaningful day and in knowing what makes life special to her. When we can frame her day to make her feel successful, the enrichment to her life will be abundant.

For instance, consider the following as a start to a plan of care for Rose.

Knowing Rose likes to wake early, we want to help her to do so. She will also like going to bed early. Rose values a good breakfast. Allowing her to help fix breakfast would make her feel useful.

It is important to identify meals by using the words that Rose knows – **dinner** at noontime, and **supper** in the early evening.Involving Rose with setting the table and cleaning up afterward will be important to her.Mid-morning might be a good time to involve Rose in folding laundry, or watering the garden.Rose will probably be more interested in the noon meal than in the evening meal. Making this the bigger meal of the day is a way to provide success for Rose.The evening meal should be a light snack, sandwich, soup or salad. Rose will most likely feel worth when she is helping to prepare the food. She may need encouragement and praise for reassurance, but this will mean a lot to her.As Rose sits at the window, reminisce with her about farm days. Ask her what crop is being planted now. Discuss the weather and how it may affect the fields. Ask her questions about farming and how the men worked.

Can you find other clues from Rose's life to add value to her day? There are plenty more, it just takes creativity, time and patience. When we understand the life story of a person with memory impairment, life becomes a whole lot easier. We can go to their world and help them have a good day. Remember, a person with dementia cannot relate and adjust to our world, so we must adjust and relate to theirs. This concept alone will completely change the way you interact. It will make you very successful, too. By reading their facial signals, sensing the hunger signs that you learn from their biography, and appealing to them with their favorite food and drink, served in that personal way, the life of your memory impaired person can become very, very good. And in turn, your life is getting better - the payoff is beginning to happen! Time is becoming your friend and you are both having a better day.

CHAPTER 3

REKINDLING THE STORY WITHIN

When you think of mealtimes in your own past, what are the warm and familiar thoughts that come to mind?

In my own life, I think about the way we all six sat down to supper together. We had a standard prayer before dinner that went like this:

Bless us, o Lord, for these thy gifts, which we are about to receive, from all thy bounty. Through Christ our Lord, Amen. If were very hungry, or it was a favorite meal, the prayer seems to be spoken quickly. I smile as remember my younger brother Pat, who was always ravenous, and how he would race through the prayer to get to his food. This memory makes me smile.

Then there is the memory of the lazy susan we had in the middle of our farm table. It was big and held the dishes of food to be shared. We would each have a hand on the edge of the wheel in front of us. Grabbing and spinning... sometimes shaking the food dishes nearly off the spindle! Mom would scowl and Dad would grin. We would then continue on, waiting our turn so we would not be scolded.

Another memory is of the barbeques we used to have, inviting friends or relatives to come and share a Sunday afternoon. We had a swimming pool, and so it was a perfect gathering spot. Dad would BBQ, Mom would make potato salad, and we each got to turn the crank on the ice cream maker. Those barbequed hamburgers never tasted as good as after a afternoon of swimming and sunning.

As I got older and lived on my own, those food memories became even more precious to me. I would return home on the weekends to swim and have a barbequed meal. We would sit at the farm table and the lazy susan was loaded with dishes. Sometimes one of us would grab the edge and spin the lazy susan as hard as we could, just for old times sake.

As a middle age adult, there are food connections I have formed through the years that have become part of my lifestyle. The connections from my childhood are still alive, and more memories have been added along through time.

Everyone has their unique and special food memories, made strong by the emotional connections attached to these memories. When I think of how good the Thanksgiving turkey tasted each year, I reminisce about the family and friends gathered around the occasion through the years. Some years are extra special, because the emotional ties are more vivid, like the last Thansgiving my father shared with us.

The concept of emotional memory is a separate concept from cognitive or intellectual memory. Those deep bonds and feelings we carry in our heart are never broken. The names and places that we made those memories around might not be recalled, but the essence of the love that was shared and how our lives were touched never seems to leave us. This is why is it so important to pinpoint and celebrate the personal emotional memories that are inside every one of us. These emotional memories hold the key to unlocking joy and love and a new freedom that builds meaning, every bit as much for the person with dementia as for you and I. If we can recapture those moments that hold true meaning and value for us, we find a real quality about life that warms our hearts and brings true peace.

This might seem abstract, the concept of emotional memory, but I have seen these important connections made time and again with the memory impaired person. Knowing what creates the smile within and how to revive that wonderful feeling is the magic that makes life worth living.

So finding the memories that 'sparkle the eyes' becomes the key to making life happen in a new and glorious way. Just imagine how your life would be if people around you looked for ways to make you happy! Getting to the heart of who you are caring for is the first step in creating this happiness for them.

Let me give you a picture of what I mean:

Let's suppose I developed dementia and needed care support. First and foremost, I suspect I would be devastated. It would probably take some time to absorb this information. Once I was able to get my mind around the idea, there would be some fear about what will happen to me. So this is where I would start to think about what my life will look like. I am sure there would be many values that I would want people to understand about me. Here is a start:

I would want my lifestyle to be respected. And it is the same for anyone with dementia. We carry our personalities and our lifestyle right along with us when we develop memory impairment- they cannot be separated. So what would a caregiver need to know about me?

First, I am an early riser, usually up by 6:30 AM and I like coffee first thing in the morning. I would like to take a shower and then sit down to the newspaper, coffee and maybe some oatmeal. I also enjoy yogurt with blueberries on top.

Then I go about my day, with a variety of activities and tasks. I am pretty active in the morning, taking a walk, always with my dog. I love to be outside in the cool of the morning, and I enjoy the sunrise. Keep me near a window if I am inside, so I can feel the sunlight. If I am outside, I like to water, prune, cut flowers and birdwatch.

I am usually hungry by about 12:00. I like a salad for lunch, with bread. I will eat soup in the winter, but not in the summer. I will eat a sandwich if it is turkey and on wheat bread. Not white bread. I like iced tea. I don't drink milk. I like water with lemon, too. If you try to give me ham or salami or egg salad I will not eat any of those.

In the afternoon, I am more settled. I will read, or phone friends, socialize or shop. I like farmers markets. I like to shop in specialty food stores. I would really enjoy a trip to a Whole Foods Market, or someplace like that. Because I have enjoyed cooking all my life, food stores are a real treat. So are cooking stores like Williams Sonoma or Crate and Barrel. You will never hear a peep of complaint out of me if you take me to one of these places.

In the evening time, I like to be outdoors in the mild weather. I will sit outside in the yard, play with the dog and cat, and water the flowers. I love to walk.

Evening time meals are always best when barbequed for me. Especially vegetables, a rib eye steak, and grilled french bread. In the winter months, I enjoy soup and a salad. My favorite desserts are butter pecan ice cream, fresh strawberries, or chocolate.

I like to settle in for a movie at home with popcorn and snuggle under an afghan on the couch. If I fall asleep, that's OK. I will wake up and go to bed, eventually.

So now that you have a good idea what my lifestyle is like, think of what you would like a caregiver to know about you. Imagine an ordinary day for you, and how it may look. I'll bet it is very different from the day I just described. By going through this exercise, you will have an enlightened look at seeing through the eyes of your memory impaired friend.

To gather information, ask many questions of all family members. If this is a spouse, take out old photographs and reminisce together. You may be surprised how much you learn! Photographs can hold the key to many cherished connections and can provide a way to rekindle special times past. When they revolve around food, they become even more cherished.

A RECIPE TO SHARE

Old-fashioned Peach Buckle

Serves 8 – Prep time 15 minutes – total time 60 minutes

This great favorite is baked in a cast iron skillet, and served right out of the skillet. If you don't have one available, use a 9" square baking pan. Again, serve this straight from the pan.

½ C (one stick) unsalted butter, softened, plus a little more for the skillet
¾ C + 2 Tablespoons sugar

3 large eggs
1 teaspoon vanilla extract
1 ¼ C Flour
½ teaspoon baking powder
½ teaspoon salt
4 C total peaches, peeled, and cut into ½"
pieces (any other fruit can be substituted)
1 teaspoon ground cinnamon
½ C walnuts, sliced almonds, or pecans

Preheat oven to 350 degrees F. Butter a 10" or
larger cast iron skillet.
In a large bowl, cream butter and ¾ C sugar
with an electric mixer until fluffy.

Add the eggs one at a time, and the vanilla.
Beat to combine.
In a medium bowl, whisk together the flour,
baking powder and salt.
With the mixer on low speed, gradually add
the flour mixture to the butter mixture.
Beat togther until well blended.
Fold in your peaches or other fruit.
Spread your batter into the skillet.
In a small bowl, combine the remaining 2 T
sugar, the cinnamon and the nuts.

Sprinkle this mixture over the top of the batter.
Place skillet in oven, uncovered.
Bake until a toothpick inserted in center comes out clean, and the top of the buckle is golden.
Total baking time is around 45-55 minutes.
Let buckle cool 20 minutes before serving.
Cut wedges out of the skillet, and top with vanilla ice cream, if you like.

BUILDING A PERSONAL FOOD 'ALBUM'

Questions to ask:
What is your favorite drink in the summer? In the winter? (Describe a hot/cold day and ask)
Did you visit your grandmother's house when you were young? What kinds of foods did she fix? Did you have a favorite?
When you were growing up, what was your favorite treat?
Did your mother bake pies?
What was your favorite holiday meal?
Did you enjoy grocery shopping? Did you have a favorite cereal?
Tell me about your birthday dinners. How did you celebrate and what would you ask for?
Did your mother cook for you?
What was dinnertime like in your house?

Did your spouse help in the kitchen?
Did you come from a big family, and was everyone at the table together?
Do you like/did you like to cook or grill?
What is your favorite meal?
Do you like spicy food – like Mexican or Chinese?
Did you eat out much? If so, where did you like to go, and what did you eat?

Some of these questions may be appropriate, and some may be too difficult for the person with memory impairment to answer. Keep in mind the abilities your person still has. Get your questions answered by other family members as you can. The more you can learn about the individual tastes, rhythms, and lifestyle of your memory impaired person, the quicker you will be able to meet their needs and give them a pleasureable dining experience.

CHAPTER 4

SETTING THE TABLE FOR SUCCESS

This is where the scene is produced. We have done our homework , gathered stories, preferences, values, and we feel like we understand what our memory impaired person needs, and what aspects of mealtime are important to them. Now to put this information into action. Here are a few general guidelines to help make your dining table a memorable experience.

AMBIENCE

This involves the whole environment, starting with background noise, such as the TV, radio, computer, whatever may be adding to the noise level. Make sure that all this noise is eliminated. The only exception here is that if your person tends to become agitated or anxious easily, you may want to play some very soft, soothing music, set at a low volume for comfort.

LIGHTING

The lighting is a big factor in ambience. The stronger and brighter the light, the better, especially toward the evening meal. Persons with dementia can tend to experience high levels of agitation later in the day (known as sundowning), and this is directly related to the amount of shadows and the natural sunlight dimming at the end of day – which is why the behavior is called sundowning. Research has shown that by keeping a high level of light in the home, this can decrease agitation due to the improved sense of vision. Again, you will want to make sure that there is plenty of light over the table. One key to keep in mind – those flourenscent, low-watt bulbs that cast a strange light are known to be agitating. Use soft white bulbs in your lighting. Or best yet, eat by natural light if this fits in with the person's values.

Some people like to use candles to create ambience. I would discourage this, not only for safely reasons, but because candles can seem frightening to a person with dementia.

In setting the table, try to use a tablemat or placemat that has a plain but contrasting color to the dishware. This will provide extra cueing to the eye, and allow the person to see where their place setting begins and ends. The best type of dishware to use is solid in color, without print or design. This is because a design can be confused with food, and often the person may be trying to scrape at the pattern on a plate, thinking it is food. A lip or edge to a plate is helpful to contain food also.

Square tables will be more comforting and secure than round tables. This is due to the fact that people with dementia feel a sense of security when they know where their 'borders' lie. This can be established by a square table much easier. I have seen persons reach over to the next plate, thinking they have their own, when sitting at a round table.

Using the minimal silverware possible for the meal is best, and keeping the utensils limited to what is needed for the meal at hand is advised. Also, serve just one beverage glass at a time. If you are serving juice and water, for example, serve the water first,and once it is finished, follow with the juice.

When serving several courses, like soup, salad and entrée, break these down by serving one course at a time, and clear the course when finished. Then serve the next one, and so on. If we allow several courses to sit in front of the person at once, this creates confusion and might make the person stop eating altogether. (Known as over-stimulation, we can cause frustration by trying to accommodate all senses at once.)

It may be that you can ask your person to help you by setting the table, or by pouring beverages, and if so, please enlist in their help. This will provide interest in the meal, and help them to feel useful at the same time. This technique can be done after the meal also. If they are able to help you, let them. They may be slow, awkward, or clumsy, but that's alright. The point is, they are participating and feel engaged in the activity. Fill a sink with soapy water, and allow them to soak the dishes. It makes no matter that you have a dishwasher- you can always fill it later. The ability to contribute to the meal is a responsibility that many older folk feel obliged to take. Let them.

I worked with a man named Phil who had never spent any time in the kitchen. He was a fighter pilot in World War II and had many stories to tell. Once the war ended, he came back to his hometown and married, and settled down on a farm. Often times, he would have illusions that his plane had been hit, and that he needed to respond. This would lead to a full-blown anxiety attack, and his caregivers were beside themselves with panic about how to calm him down. The last year, as his dementia became more involved, Phil lost his interest in food. He has no desire to eat and was losing weight. Getting him involved in the kitchen was next to impossible. Phil did not engage in household chores, because in his mind, his wife took care of all that. This case became a tall order, and something had to be done, and quick.

Phil had one interest- his tractor. He babied his Ford tractor like it was a son – the son he never had. He talked about the tractor and spent a lot of time tinkering with it. Phil had not used the tractor in years, the farm had been set up in pasture and there was no need to cultivate.

One day I asked Phil to help me with some equipment. I had a commercial dishwasher that you would find in a restaurant kitchen – and I needed him to look at it for me. He was very hesitant and unphased. He was not about to look at something that he knew nothing about. But something told me to persist. When I was able to get him to walk to the kitchen with me and showed him the mechanics of this machine – the vertical sliding door and the toggle switches that controlled the power, drain basin, water level fill, and temperature gauges, his attitude changed. He began to study the parts and makeup of the machine, lifting the door and trying out the switches. Now there was not anything wrong with the machine, but that was not the point. Phil now was asking questions and experimenting with this new-found equipment. Once I showed him how it worked and let him know that whatever he did, it worked, he was pleased. Now that I had his attention, I gave him a thank you gift- a bowl of soup and a sandwich. I sat him down near the dishwasher and asked him to let me do the work. Loading the dishwasher and putting it through a short cycle, Phil could watch the process from his seat, while eating. Before we knew it, the dishes were done and Phil was done with his meal, too. Phil felt worth, success, and warmth from 'fixing' the machine and connecting with another person in a meaningful way.

Once the meal is finished, this is a good time to take a short walk, if possible. If this is not an option, use the wheelchair to get some fresh air together. Afterward, it is amazing how refreshed you both will feel.

CHAPTER 5

FOOD PUZZLES

When looking at the overall picture, putting together the dementia 'puzzle' will be the starting point to find the solutions needed to make meals work well. Here are some puzzle pieces that may help in discovering the whole picture.

First – determine what the person can do for themselves. Here's a scenario to start us off:

Emily is caring for Anne, an 80 year old woman who is diagnosed with early stage Alzheimer's disease. Anne has been living alone, but her daughter who looks in on her twice a day has noticed that she is not eating much. The meals that are brought in for her are ending up un-eaten in the fridge, or mistakenly placed in the freezer (by Anne). Although she is losing weight, the other areas of her life seem manageable to her family. Anne can get dressed independently in the morning, she takes care of her personal hygiene, and she is fairly pleasantly confused most of the time. Anne usually accepts direction, although she does not initiate activity on her own. If left alone, Anne will sit in a chair, watch TV, flip through magazines, and possibly putter around the house. She rarely diplays emotional outbursts, but she can become frustrated when Emily asks her to complete multi-step activities. Anne is not very interested in eating or drinking much. She is about eight to ten pounds under her usual weight of 135 pounds.

Emily's day involves cleaning, laundry, meals for Anne, taking her to doctor appointments and general supervision. When she can, Emily plans a fun activity to do together, although Anne is not very enthusiastic. Mealtime usually takes quite a while, since Emily must spend a great deal of time getting Anne interested in eating.

How can we help Emily?

First of all, we need more information about Anne, don't we? Let's ask her daughter more about her. Recall the questions in Chapter 2 and build a list that you would like her daughter to answer. This will be your puzzle frame. Once you have the frame, you can begin to fill in with your own approaches.

By involving Anne in the meal preparation, she has the opportunity to feel needed, and this creates a meaningful time for Anne. When we create emotional meaning for a person with dementia, there is a connection taking place. The more connections, the better the sense of well-being for the memory impaired. Meaningful times then equal more motivation, which in turn equals happier moments.

Here's how we could find out what Anne can do, and how to make things easier for Emily:

Invite Anne to help in the kitchen. Start with a simple task- washing vegetables for dinner. Offer simple, step-by-step instruction that she can process. Watch her respond to you, and slow down if you need to. Remember that the object is connecting, and the quality of the connection. If Anne succeeds, see if she would like to peel a potato – and so forth. Be sure to check her body language, as she may feel as though this is enough for her. If so, don't push. Just thank her and praise her for the great job she did. Anne may feel awkward or clumsy, yet by reassuring her, she will continue. If she appears frustrated, simply allow her to stop, and then change the focus. Maybe just ask her to sit and watch. Since this may be all she can handle - that's OK. No worries! The important thing is that she is taking part, even by observing! It is amazing what can happen in the soul by being included in the meal process.

Depending on how long Anne will stay involved, Emily might ask her to help set the table. This may be done by role modeling and allowing her to mimic the action. Set one place at the table, and give Anne the utensils to complete another place setting. See what happens.

By taking activities in small, simple steps, the memory impaired person has a much better chance of succeeding, which translates to enjoying, what is happening. This exercise allows for a 'test pattern' of Anne's abilities, and those abilities are then duplicated in other activities. We have now created a template for success!

But you say, that sounds too easy. So let's take another spin on the situation:

Anne might feel motivated to help more than Emily wants. Now what? By constructively steering Anne in a way that uses her energy productively, Emily can put the 'action' to good use. Maybe it's filling ice cube trays, or scrubbing the kitchen sink, or arranging flowers for the table while you are cooking. Try to give her something to do that will make her feel like she is involved and important.

Or, suppose this is the case:

Emily has just a short amount of time to get breakfast ready before she has to take Anne to the doctor. In this case, Emily can ask Anne to help her by sitting down. Then while Emliy is preparing breakfast, Anne can peel her banana and start on that. She may begin with cereal and milk, or a cup of yogurt.

If we can keep things in perspective, make the situation work in everyone's favor, life will be so much easier and the memory impaired person will feel much more relaxed.

EMOTIONAL MIRRORING

The most important area of cooperation that seems to escape most caregivers is the area of emotional mirroring. When a memory impaired person is acting out, we often cannot figure out why. There seems to be no reason for their behavior.

One reason could be that we are projecting our emotional state onto them, without realizing it. If we just received a call from the bank and there has been a mixup with a deposit, it is natural to feel upset and bothered, possibly angry with the bank. The memory impaired person cannot understand your emotions and the only way they know to react is to mirror your feelings. So we now have two upset, bothered and angry people. The issue is now compounded for you, the caregiver, and that is NOT what you need!

A word to the wise on this situation: when giving care, the best thing we can do as caregivers is to leave our stress buttons somewhere else. The more peaceful a setting we can provide, the smoother time we will enjoy – which in turn brings our external stressors back under control. Everyone is better off!

LET'S TAKE A LOOK AT ANOTHER SCENARIO:

Bob and Betty have been married 61 years. Bob has been in sales his entire career. Betty has raised 4 children and prides herself on her homemaking abilities – she bakes, quilts, gardens, puts up canned vegetables, and keeps an immaculate home.

Bob was diagnosed with Alzheimer's Disease three years ago. His personality is shifting: he knows that he has Alzheimer's, and this is very upsetting to him. Bob has begun to isolate himself from his friends, he no longer feels confident about his golf game, and he prefers to sit in front of the TV and sulk.

Betty is heartbroken to see her husband in such a state and wants to help, but Bob resents Betty for what he considers 'nagging' at him. He hardly touches his meals, and snacks on potato chips and ice cream in his recliner instead, which frustrates Betty. Because Bob is gregarious in nature, he becomes irate when Betty prompts him to the dinnertable. Many times an argument will begin, at which point Bob decides he is not giving in and goes without his meal. Betty is distraught and both spend the evening in silence.

WHAT CAN BE DONE HERE?

To start, Bob is probably depressed. He may need to see his doctor, to see if an anti-depressant might help. This can be a very tricky time, what we call the "I know that I don't know" stage. It is very difficult, especially for men, to be going through this stage. Due to his role as head of the house, Bob needs to feel that he is still in control, that he is still capable of making decisions, and that his decisions are needed by Betty. This concept is key. By giving Bob choices that require a decision on his part, Bob can maintain that feeling of control. The decisions don't have to be big ones, just choices that Bob can make that help him feel like he is still in charge.

If Betty will ask Bob, "What would you like me to prepare for dinner Bob, meatloaf, or chicken, the way you like it over rice?" Betty may find that Bob will appreciate the chance to make his choice. Once he has, Betty can ask him for help in small ways, possibly to mix the meatloaf for her (she can complain of a sore finger or wrist) or maybe he can peel potatoes for her.

Betty may find that by being useful, this helps Bob to regain his self-worth. By nature, men are defined by their work, on an individual and collective basis. When we give them meaningful work to do that makes them feel needed, it fills that value for them. Also, we can help create a whole new emotional connection for them.

Bob may want to make a salad, or help with the dishes. Even though this has always been Betty's work, Bob can be made to feel helpful to her by the invitation to help. Asking Bob to open jars and cans for Betty is a natural. Betty can even intentionally tighten them and plead for a stronger hand.

So, we get Bob involved, but when it's time to eat, he says, I'm not hungry. Now what? Here are some ideas:

- How about offering to rub his feet after dinner?

- Invite Bob to just share a salad with you, after all, you don't want to eat alone...

- Make a quick brown sauce (from a package) and invite Bob to partake now, apologizing that you completely forgot how much he likes gravy on his meatloaf...

- Allow Bob to go sit down and let him rest. Reapproach him in 15 minutes. Chances are he will reconsider.

- Remind Bob that you made his favorite dish, as he instructed you.

- Tempt him with his favorite ice cream – if he will finish his meal (or even part of it).

- Try some roasted nuts, such as almonds for an appetizer. He will become thirsty and this might bring him to the table.

- By making the meal the important event for Bob, we revisit that instinct that has never left him, just may be buried deeper now.

Of course we realize that food is a really big deal for men - all men. I have never run across a man, memory impaired or otherwise, that does not respond well to food, especially meat and potatoes! Just talking about food can be a great activity. By using magazines and cookbooks with pictures, men can be enticed to select foods that they would enjoy eating. There is another great way to complete the puzzle. Grocery shopping is one activity that could work, but this needs to be measured and on a limited basis at a slow time of day. Do not try to shop with your memory impaired person on a Saturday! This could be a recipe for disaster. Grocery stores are full of stimulation, so if you attempt this activity, have an organized list and lots of patience.

CHAPTER 6

BALANCING THE NUTRITION TIGHTROPE

Alright, we all remember something about the food pyramid. And you have been taught about a balanced diet, three square meals a day, and that it is necessary to eat your vegetables. Now that you are caring for someone with memory impairment, all the rules seem to suddenly go out the window, don't they?

It seems like no matter how hard you try to make sure that you are preparing a nutritious, healthy meal, all your efforts sometimes can go down the drain (literally!). Either they pick at the food, they aren't hungry, or the vegetables and fruit go completely untouched. This can be very frustrating, to say the least.

For many older adults, the issue of appetite can be a tricky one. To begin with, older adults need fewer calories a day to get by. This is because they are typically burning less energy, but not all people are alike, right? So how do we know when someone is getting enough to eat? Many times a person may say, "I'm just not hungry" and that may truly be how they feel. But that doesn't mean that they don't need to replenish their energy stores.

With dementia, many times the area of the brain that tells us when we are hungry does not function properly. It may be missing signals, which means there could be no appetite stimulation going on at all. This is the most challenging of instances. Here we need to get real creative and look at inviting sensory tools to the table. Foods with strong aromas, lots of texture, bright colors, and a lot of flavor might be the best approach.

So how much food does an older adult need each day? Here is a basic and general guideline for adults over 60 years old:

5-6 ounces of protein (meat, fish, eggs)
6-11 servings of breads and cereal
5 servings of fruit and vegetables

2 servings of dairy products
Total intake: about 1800-2000 calories a day

You may be thinking, "Good Grief! That's a lot of food!" Now let me clarify – the serving size is ½ cup for breads, cereals, fruit, and vegetables. The protein serving is just as big as a deck of cards, and if you are using eggs, it translates to 2 whole eggs. When we consider what most Americans think of as a portion, especially by restaurant standards, it is astounding to realize that we are typically eating 5–6 portions in one helping! Did you ever look at an order of 'super-size fries'? This is typically 4 servings, and not even close to healthy for anyone to consume!

Most Americans cover 2 servings of bread/cereal and 2 servings of milk when they eat a bowl of Wheaties in the morning. That's a great way to start the day.

An egg salad sandwich, for example, contains 2 servings of bread, one serving of protein, and one vegetable (if you add lettuce and tomato).

A dinner consisting of spagetti with meat sauce, green salad and garlic bread would cover 3 bread/cereal servings, 2 vegetable servings, 1 meat serving, and depending on the salad ingredients, maybe one more vegetable serving.

So you see the daily intake can add up fast, and if we are able to give the right combinations of food, we can keep the nutritional balance in check.

The biggest area of concern for most folks is the fruit and vegetables. Think about this: 5 servings can be covered in one nice tasty garden salad. If we look at adding shredded cheese and diced ham, you are covering a dairy and half a protein serving (or more if you pile it on).

Think creatively when you are looking at preparing from the recommended daily allowances for older adults (RDA's). Here are a few sample menus for you to try out. Mix and match them according to individual taste and preferences.

BREAKFAST

Cereal and Milk
1 piece of toast
1 fruit
coffee

Oatmeal w/raisins
Muffin
1 fruit
fruit juice

French Toast
Bacon
1 fruit milk

Pancakes
Sausage links
1 fruit
Milk

Bagel and cream cheese
1 fruit
Milk or juice

Belgian Waffles
Ham slice

1 fruit
coffee

Biscuits and gravy
Bacon
1 fruit
Milk

Cheese Omelet
Sausage links
1 fruit
juice

These ideas can work at one meal time, or can be served in two smaller meals. Use your food connection clues to see what works best. The key is to ask, observe and implement.

When one or two ideas are working really well, it is important to stick with them. A person with memory impairment lives best by routine and structure. If you develop a routine in the morning and serve the 'winners' you will have a much smoother day ahead.

Sometimes introducing a new food is confusing and can disorient a person. If you are trying something new, the best approach is to sit down with the person and describe what you are serving them. Then ask permission to sit down and enjoy that meal with them. Many times the idea goes over much easier if you can show that you are giving them something you would enjoy yourself – and then continue to share the meal together. The notion of "mirroring" what you are eating is a great way to get them started.

FLUIDS

Lets talk about the stuff that 80% of our bodies are made of – water. This vital fluid is often overlooked as we go about our care giving day. We find that those with dementia just don't seem to want liquids. This is understandable, mainly because most older adults have a decreased sense of thirst. This decrease in thirst is due to the glands that produce saliva, which are slowing down. When we don't salivate as much, we don't realize we are thirsty. Also, one symptom of dementia is loss of thirst. The brain has lost the message signal from the body that there is a need for hydration.

However, the organs know when they are lacking fluids. The body responds by beginning to take fluids from vital areas, such as muscle tissue, and that includes the brain. A dehydrated person may become weak, prone to stumble and fall. This is clearly a sign of dehydration. Also, when a person with dementia becomes increasingly confused, or out of sorts, there could be dehydration going on. Offer some fluids, water, juice or iced tea right away. Give them a few hours rest and see if that doesn't help. Often the body needs time to reabsorb the fluids it is missing before rebalancing itself.

So what is the best way to make sure a person with dementia has enough liquids on a daily basis?

First of all, what is 'enough'? That will be different as it relates to body size, age, and lifestyle. If we look at a general amount, six 8-ounce glasses, or 48 ounces in a day is probably a good average. When we consider a large man, who may walk a lot during the day, he may need 8–10 glasses of water. A petite woman with a quiet routine, that is to say just the minimal amount of exercise, may on require just five glasses a day.

Once we look at the person and their activity level, the goal would be to encourage water or fluids throughout the day, to meet the overall daily goal. This can be approached in several ways. A glass of juice with a meal is great. A glass of water after a walk is good timing. Keeping the portions to 4–6 ounces at a time is less overwhelming to a person who doesn't believe they are thirsty, than a 8–10 ounce glass of fluid. You stand a much better chance of getting two 4-ounce glasses down than one 8 ounce glass. When asking the person to drink, if you hand the glass to them, reaching out and asking them to take it, this instantly starts the process of hand to mouth. It is simple and seems overstated, but it works! By setting a glass down in front of a person, we are now asking them to make the decision to drink. This becomes another step in the process, and many times that glass never leaves the table! So try the hand-off technique and see how that works for you.

A word here about the type of fluids: the best thing to drink is water, of course. Next best is fruit juice, preferably 100% fruit juice. Watch labels because many 'fruit juices' actually contain little to no juice, and instead are filled with sugar and flavorings. The next best thing is herbal tea. These can be made at home, and can be an 'activity' to do together, especially herbal sun teas.

Stay away from caffeinated drinks, like coffee, tea and soda pop. These contain acids that may be sensitive to their stomach, and these beverages tend to have a dehydrating quality also, which works against you- for every cup of coffee consumed, the body needs a cup of water to replace the fluids the coffee is drawing out of the system.

Another helpful hint: Keep a pitcher of water on the counter, filled with ice, and slice an orange or lemon or lime and float this in the top of the pitcher. It will make for a nice flavor, will look interesting, and the visual cue will prompt the person to try it. Keep a small size cup or two sitting next to the pitcher, so as to provide for visual cueing.

KIM'S REFRESHER

1 C Pineapple Juice
1 C Cranberry Juice
2 C Ginger Ale
½ teaspoon almond extract
Ice

Mix all together in a pitcher and serve over ice.
Will keep for a day.

CHAPTER 7

NEVER FEAR, HELP IN NEAR!

We've created the best climate possible for your memory impaired person to enjoy their meal . Sometimes the best laid plans can go sideways, without a moment's warning. Let's take a look at a couple of issues that you may be experienceing in your caregiving:

PACING – NOT WANTING TO SIT DOWN

This is a very common trait for people with Alzheimer's Disease. The mind is searching, processing and wanting to gather a sense of security. This is seen through fidgeting, repetitive motions, and wanting to get somewhere they believe they need to be.

This is a difficult issue to address, since the person must be distracted off of their 'mind path' and brought into a new realm, which is the meal you have prepared. Leaving the person to do as they please will only postphone the meal until later, which doesn't help to get the nutrition delivered. Here you may want to give the person a sandwich and place it in their hand. This allows for a win-win situation. Many times the person will take a bite and set it down. That's OK. Just offer it again. By placing a finger food into the palm of the hand, a person can have the flexibility to roam around and take a bite as they please. A word of caution here: food can be set down and left in strange places – I have known folks to find a partially eaten apple, sandwich or other food in a dresser drawer, a bathroom cabinet or a flower bed.

DISINTEREST IN EATING

This is one issue that faces nearly all caregivers at one time or another. We can see that no matter what we do, the person just has no desire to sit down at the table, much less to begin to enjoy their food. There could be many reasons for this behavior, and we can discuss them in detail.

One reason could be the medications that are being taken. For instance, Aricept has a pronounced side effect of decreased appetite. There is also a side effect for some folks of diarrhea. So between these two effects, there is lttle chance that someone would have an appetite.

Another reason is the visual presentation of the food. We know that we all eat with our eyes and our nose before we do our mouth. The more appealing the food looks, the more desire to eat. Also, aromas make a big difference. Bringing the person into the kitchen and asking them to smell the food, and help stir or taste it for you gives them an opportunity to be involved, smell the food, and arouse their interest. Sometimes just the act of helping out can bring back the intuitive role of mealtime, and the meal can flow forward much easier.

Again, these are just two areas of potential change. What about the notion that a memory impaired person just has no desire to sit down to the table, despite your efforts? There are a couple more things you may want to try. First, try serving the meal in courses, even breaking down the meat, veggies and starch by serving each in a separate, small dish or plate. A person with dementia can become overwhelmed quite easily, and by simplifying the meal this can reduce the anxiety that might come on by sitting down to a full plate of foods that the person may not feel comfortable in trying to begin consuming.

Here is another thought – keeping it simple, which can mean removing any condiments, salt, pepper, vases, fluff or anything else on the table that might be distracting. If we consider the amount of focus that may be necessary for the person to complete a meal, we surely want them to feel minimally affected by a table full of items that might overwhelm.

To get a person's taste buds going, smelling something good in the kitchen does the trick. If your meal is such that the food you are preparing doesn't necessarily have an aroma, try this: about an hour before mealtime, place a sliced onion with a couple of garlic cloves in a baking pan and place this in a 375 degree oven. The aroma that develops is like a roast cooking, and this trick also will have the neighbors salivating. After an hour, remove the onion and garlic and they can always be used in a sauce or soup.

Another trick is to put together a mulled cider and have that simmering on the stove. This is a great wintertime activity that can be done together. Here's how:

Take 2 quarts of apple cider and place in a saucepot.
Add the following:
Two cinnamon sticks
One orange, quartered and studded with 3 cloves in each orange quarter
2 -6 sugar cubes, sweetening to taste
Now bring the above items to a slow simmer over medium heat. Remove the spices and orange quarters. Serve in coffee mugs. This beverage can be served with the meal and later for a nice treat.

PLAYING WITH THE FOOD

Here again we first think about keeping everything simple. This is also a behavior that can be modified through role modeling. When you sit down to eat with the person, you provide a mirror for them to follow. Sometimes serving the beverage after the majority of the meal is finished is a good way to motivate the person toward the food and not the drink. I have seen memory impaired pour the milk over their plate of food and then wonder what has happened. Of course this is nonsense to us, but can create much confusion to the person. Also, take a look at how the person may or may not be using their utensils. Often times we see that a fork becomes a foreign object that is hard to manipulate. A spoon or tablespoon may work better. See if the knife is too difficult to use - this is a clue that it is time to serve the food prepared to eat from one untensil, like the Chinese do. Cutting up food at the table is discouraged, as this can be seen as demeaning. We would do better to present the food in a ready-to-eat manner, which preserves the person's dignity.

SPITTING OUT OR POCKETING FOOD

Sometimes the food is taken easily, but in the chewing process, the person decides to part with the food. Spitting out food usually means that the texture seems odd, or that the food is too dry. If we place a sauce over the meat, or make sure there is butter on the potatoes or bread, that provides a juicier food that is easier to swallow. Because older adults lose saliva as they age, the need for additional wetting agents becomes important. The juicier, the better!

Pocketing food has to do with chewing and forming a bolus or ball to swallow, and then placing that bolus inside the lower cheek and never swallowing it. The person may continue to eat and never swallow, all the while accumulating a chipmunk-like appearance due to the storage of food. Again, we want to watch the person if they are not swallowing each bite, offer a liquid to help wash the bolus down, or remind the person that the food is there by gently massaging the cheek. This may seem odd, but if a person is pocketing food, they will be unaware that it is there, and you will be keeping them from choking by pushing that food back toward the tongue.

Another reason food may be spit out is that the ability to chew has become decreased through poor fitting dentures, or teeth that are in need of repair. Try to look into the mouth for sores, tender spots, sensitivity, or dentures that are rubbing on a gumline. Also, be sure that teeth aren't affected by hot or cold liquids, which is a sign of cavities or a cracked tooth.

SWALLOWING DIFFICULTIES

This problem is one that needs to be addressed just as soon as you notice it. Choking, coughing, sputtering and wheezing during eating are all signals that there could be a problem. The memory impaired person may have forgotten how to swallow. In this case, we need to have a swallowing evaluation performed by a licensed professional, ordered by the primary care physician. In many cases, the solution will be to prepare beverages using a thickening agent that will make the liquid heavier and easier to swallow. Because choking and aspirating on food is a precurser to pnemonia, this one issue that must be handled quickly. If you notice this happening, and the person has a mouthful of food, massage the throat and neck of the person in an attempt to get the swallowing mechanism started. Or it may be safer to ask them to spit the food out. Try a milkshake, a smoothie, cream soup, or something of a thicker consistency until you get them to the doctor.

EATING WITH FINGERS

This behavior is very common with memory impairment. It really only signals that the person has become more comfortable in eating with their hands instead of utensils. Let them be. You would much rather see this habit than to have them not eat. When this stage appears, it will be important to serve foods that are easier to manage with the hands.

Listed below are some ideas for 'finger foods' that can also be used for persons who prefer to eat on the go.

Hamburgers, cut in half - garden burger - deviled eggs - soup, served in a mug - tea sandwiches - stuffed pita bread - raw or cooked baby carrots - broccoli spears - cauliflower flowerettes - zucchini sticks - cheese cubes – grapes - bananas - apple slices – figs – dates - peach slices - any sliced meat, wrapped in a flour tortilla- french toast sticks – melon slices –celery with peanut butter – cherry tomatoes – cheese and crackers – french fries – tater tots – yogurt, with diced fruit or granola – popcorn – chex mix – chips and salsa – pizza – and so on.

Here are some on-the-go snacks that work very well for persons preferring to use their hands:

Place these items in a baggie: pretzels, crackers, mixed nuts, trail mix, raisins, popcorn, chilled raw veggies, fruit wedges, sliced salami and cheese cubes, pitted olives, granola and power bars, cut up into thin slices.

HAND-OVER-HAND FEEDING

Here is another option to help support the use of utensils, if it seems like the person still wants to try to use them. Start by loading the spoon or fork with food and then place the utensil in the person's hand, helping to form a grip around the handle. Then allow them to take the food to the mouth. If they are having trouble, assistance can help guide the hand to the mouth. Allowing the memory impaired person to be as independent as possible is key. This will keep them interested in eating far longer than if everything is done for them.

SCREAMING OR FUSSING

This can happen when there is too much stimulation at mealtime. For instance, if someone is working in the kitchen while the meal is going on, or there is activity or commotion in a nearby room. The best solution is to have a peaceful home where all that is happening is the meal itself. This will help keep things calm. Another upsetting activity is talking on the phone during a meal. This can bring about agitation because the person with dementia might not realize that you are not talking to them. As much as possible, try to have a quiet and calm table. It might be helpful to comment on the flavors of the food, chat about the last time you had meatloaf (if that's what is served) and make small talk about the meal itself. Anything to keep the mood light and focused is going to be helpful.

CHAPTER 8

SAVING THE BEST FOR LAST

MEET SWEET TOOTH SALLY

Here is a story about a gal I know that has an abundance of energy, morning, noon and night. Sally has Alzheimer's Disease, was diagnosed 2 years ago and is taking Aricept. She lives at home with her daughter, Linda, who is caring for her. This is what Sally's life is like now: by most scales, Sally is fairly high functioning and independent. She can still take a shower independently, dress herself, manage household tasks (with some assistance) and she likes to garden. When her daughter Linda has to go out to run errands, she feels comfortable leaving Sally alone at home for up to an hour. Sally usually just watches TV or takes a nap if Linda must leave, so this works out well.

Here is where it gets interesting. Sally likes to get up in the middle of the night to splurge on whatever sweets she can find in the house. Sally will eat ice cream, cookies, sugar cubes, jelly or jam - from the jar - and just about any other food containing sugar. She has this rationale that eating in the middle of the night makes her feel better, and so she doesn't miss too many nights. What is troubling, is that Sally is not a real good eater during the day at mealtime, and she shys away from protein, such as meat and fish. She prefers peanut butter and jelly sandwiches which help her to get her sugar fix. She will eat some fruit, but very few veggies. Sally prefers carbonated drinks and rarely will drink milk. So, you can guess there is a major issue in finding some balance to Sally's nutritional intake. How do we get a balanced diet going for Sally?

This is a very common situation for persons with early to moderate stage dementia. Initially, the brain is changing and the person is aware that things are not as they should be. This stage is the hardest, because it can lead to depression. And with depression, there comes a facet that is known as emotional eating. With emotional eating, a person tends to self-medicate with food, which brings them comfort. The most pleasurable food to a person with depression is a sugar based food. This is why we see so many early stage dementia persons craving sweets. There is a chemical called dopamine that is created in the brain's pleasure center that feeds on sugar. While the instant high is one reward, the increased dopamine in the brain makes the person feel better psychologically as well.

There are several issues going on here with Sally. If they haven't surfaced yet, they will soon enough. Sally is at high risk for becoming Type 2 diabetic. This is the first and foremost concern. With her sugar intake so high, she is sure to experience wide swings in her insulin output. Her pancreas is experiencing an overload. This can give her blood sugar the lows and highs associated with diabetes. Sally is probably feeling sluggish and sleepy during the day, due to being up at night. She will not want to eat healthy foods, as her body is set up to crave sugar and carbohydrates more than anything else. The unfortunate issue here is that Sally's body has become addicted to sugar. We know that even for a person with a healthy brain, this is a challenge to overcome. We must fight the sugar cravings and slowly wean ourselves off, and rebalance our food intake to stave off the addiction. For a person who has memory impairment, it becomes more problematic because the mind now cannot rationally process the fact that the diet needs to change. Consequently, Sally will become frustrated and possibly act out, wanting to feed the craving. Mood swings, temper outbursts, and other behaviors may soon develop.

The best way to help Sally is to get her to the doctor right away to have her tested for diabetes. Sally's doctor can then diagnose where she is and how to help manage her blood sugar levels. Linda will need to become very proactive in supervising Sally's food intake. The late night binges may take awhile to curb, and Linda may need to make other foods available to Sally that will help wean her off the sugar cravings she will still experience. By limiting the availability of sweets in the house, Sally can begin to snack on healthier items. It might be necessary to place a lock on a cupboard that contains the baking supplies. Linda would be wise to replace sugars with alternatives like fresh fruit, sugar-free cookies and snacks, and sugar-free jello and puddings. Ice cream can be replaced with fruit juice bars. If Sally has healthier options to access, chances are she will eventually transition to them.

Another solution can be to give Sally a mild sedative to help her sleep though the late night awakenings. Ask her doctor to make a recommendation. Over the counter sleep aids such as Tylenol PM have been effective to help a person sleep though the night. If a full night's sleep can be accomplished, then Sally has a good running start at the day, both from an alertness and a blood sugar standpoint.

For a person with dementia, sweets can be a huge comfort. Consider rewards and treats on a sparing level, so there is still some real quality of life and satisfaction – after all, we all like to enjoy a little sweet something now and then. In most cases, folks with dementia tend to gravitate toward sweets, especially later in the disease process. By ensuring that there is a limited quantity of healthier sweets, you are curbing the potential for an issue later on down the road.

A word about chocolate: dark chocolate contains a high antioxidant benefit. Also it contains less sugar than milk chocolate. A little dark chocolate will go a long way toward that feel-good moment.

Here are some healthier sweet-tooth ideas for snacks and desserts. Keep in mind that the average portion size for most desserts is ½ cup. (This is where almost everyone in America goes overboard!)

Trail Mix
Yogurt covered raisins or pretzels
Fresh fruit salad
Ice cream or frozen yogurt (stick with basic flavors, without chunks)
2 oatmeal cookies
Granola bar
Popcorn
Dried fruit
Whipped cream with strawberries

One very satisfying dessert is old-fashioned jello, chilled and set, that is mixed together with whipping cream (Cool-whip) and fresh cut fruit. This is a great treat. If you will use sugar-free jello, it is even healthy!

A favorite in my kitchen is a fast and easy apple crisp. Take 5 apples, core and slice them thinly. Place apples in a saucepot with ½ cup of water, 1 T lemon juice, ½ C brown sugar and 1 T cinnamon. Heat his together and then transfer mixture to a 8"x8"x2" baking dish. Then combine 2 cups of rolled whole oats with ½ C flour, ¼ C soft butter and some chopped nuts. Crumble this on the top of the apples and then bake for 30–40 minutes at 375 degrees. Serve warm with or without sugar-free ice cream. YUM!

CHAPTER 9

AFTER DINNER MINTS

The role of a caregiver is a laborious, energy-laden and emotionally draining responsibility. It has been entrusted to you, either by choice or by necessity, and you are left to accomplish the task. Entwined in all of your daily tasks of caring for your memory impaired person, is a huge demand to function as detective, nurse, social worker, and mind-reader (no pun intended). This can create an enormous amount of stress, exhaustion, overload, and burnout for you, the caregiver.

In your endeavor to deliver the best care possible, please remember the most important factor in your caregiving role: TAKING CARE OF YOU. Without the ability to rest, replenish, revive and spend time relaxing **yourself,** you will suffer more than your memory impaired person. So as you read about ways to best take care, put some of your new skills to work – on yourself. Do take the time to treat yourself to a nice meal, a candlelight dinner, a take-out meal that gives you the night out of the kitchen, and a meal out with friends. Give yourself permission to enjoy the life you work so hard to help others enjoy.

After all, you deserve to take care of you!

RECIPES

Easy Cheesy Bake

1 C cheddar cheese, grated
2 eggs, beaten
1 T butter
1 C bread crumbs
1 C milk
Salt and pepper

Preheat oven to 350 degrees. Mix all ingredients together and pout into a 8x8 baking dish. Bake for 30 minutes, or until golden brown on top.

This dish can be made together and enjoyed together - try it with some guacamole, salsa and sour cream. Or perhaps with bacon or ham.

BISCUITS AND GRAVY

Biscuits:

2 C flour
2 teaspoons baking powder
½ teaspoon cream of tartar
½ teaspoon salt
2 Tablespoons sugar
½ C shortening
2/3 C milk
1 egg

Preheat oven to 450 degrees.
In a large bowl, combine dry ingredients. Add shortening in small pieces, and blend together until crumbly. Add the milk, and then add the egg, stirring well.

Roll out the dough, dusting with flour as needed. Cut or drop by spoonfuls onto a baking sheet.

Bake for 10–15 minutes, until light brown on top.

Meanwhile...

SAUSAGE GRAVY:

¼ C butter
1 ½ pounds sausage
1 ¼ c flour
2 quarts milk
Salt and pepper

In a large skillet, melt the butter, then fry the sausage, breaking up bits and browning.

Add the flour, stirring well. Slowly add the milk, stirring as you go. Continue stirring until gravy thickens. (You may add more milk if your mixture gets too thick.) Add the seasonings to taste.

Ladle gravy over hot split biscuits. Now enjoy!

CHEF'S SALAD

2 C lettuce
1 tomato, diced
4-6 mushrooms, sliced
1 carrot, grated
¼ red onion, sliced
¼ C grated cheddar cheese
¼ C diced turkey, ham or chicken
Ranch dressing
Bacon bits – optional

Not much to putting this together, and you can do this together! I like to have your helper tear the lettuce leaves, and grate the cheese and carrots. You can even have your helper toss the salad, after you have portioned out the dressing on top.

Serve this with some warm garlic bread – healthy and satisfying.

QUICK FRUIT COBBLER

Prep time: 15 minutes Bake time: 20-30 minutes
Makes 6-8 servings

1 Can fruit pie filling – cherry, peach, blueberry,
apple or your favorite
1 C Bisquick
¼ C milk
1 Tablespoon sugar
1 Tablespoon soft butter

Spread the pie filling in an ungreased 8x8 baking dish. Place this in a cold oven. Turn the oven on the 400 degrees, and after 10 minutes, remove the pan from the oven.

While the fruit is heating, stir the remaining ingredients together until a soft dough forms. Drop this by spoonfuls onto warm pie filling. Sprinkle with additional sugar if you like.

Bake 20–25 minutes, or until the topping is light brown.

This is another simple recipe that you can engage help with. Be careful with handling the hot dish.